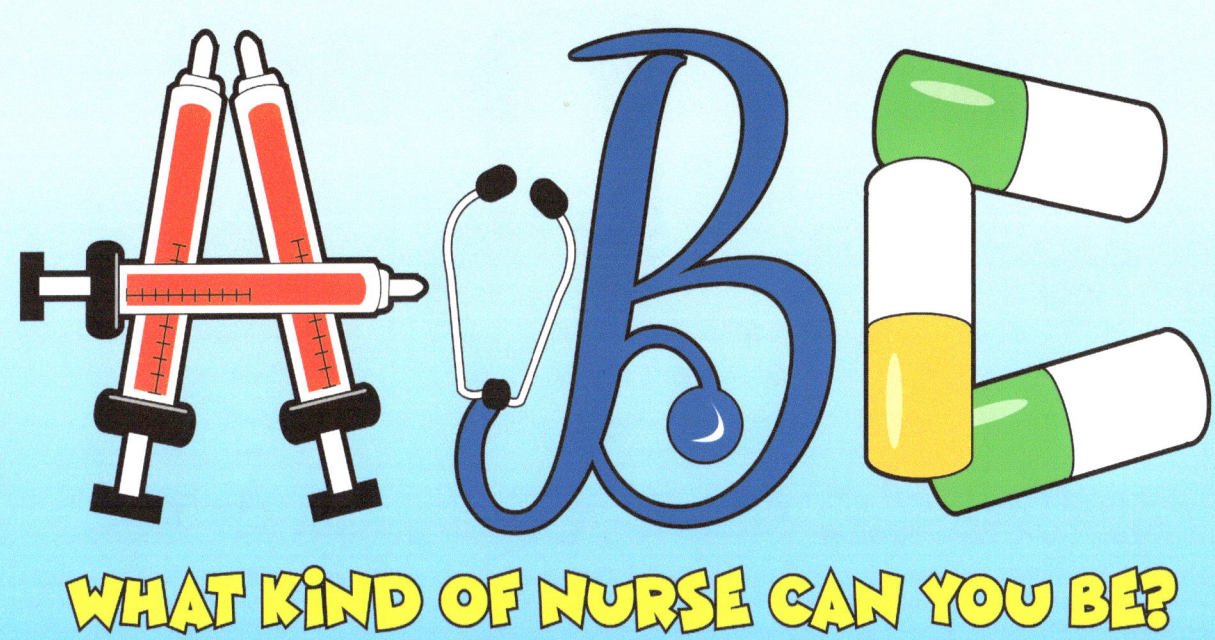

WHAT KIND OF NURSE CAN YOU BE?

Written by Cherice M. Byrd, BA, AASN
Illustrated by Kofi Johnson

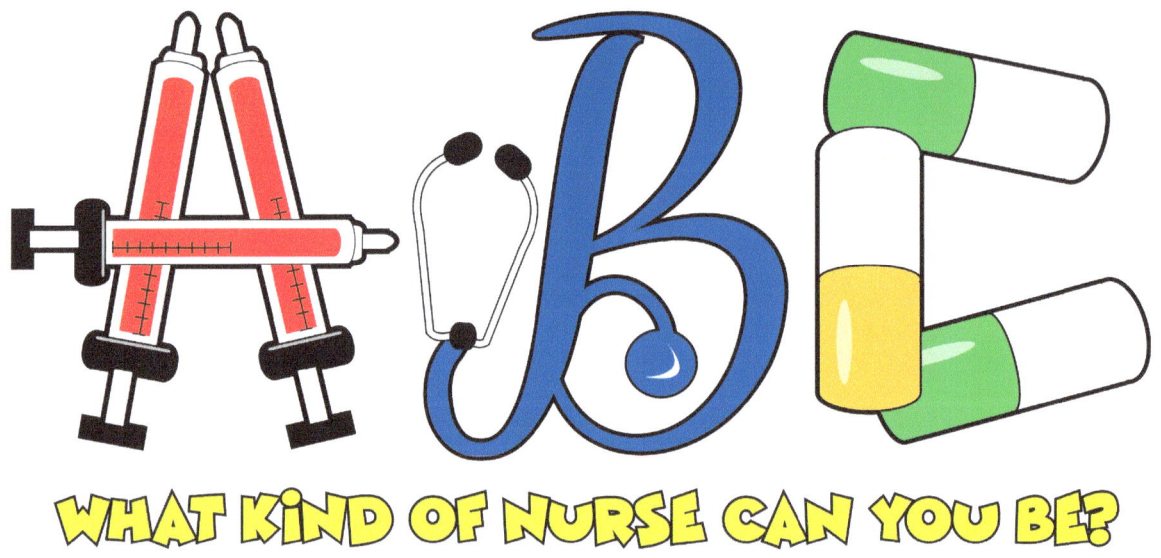

Copyright 2020 by Cherice M. Byrd, BA, AASN

All rights reserved. No part of this book may be reproduced, transmitted or stored in an information retrieval system in any form or by any means, graphic, electronic, or mechanical, including photocopying, taping, and recording without prior written permission from the author.

DEDICATION

Special thanks to my father, Jeff, for the inspiration & wisdom. To my entire incredible family for your continued love & support. For anyone who has an interest in nursing or the healthcare profession, & to all the wonderful nurses, including my phenomenal mother, Alicia, who are on the front lines that treat & care for our sick loved ones.

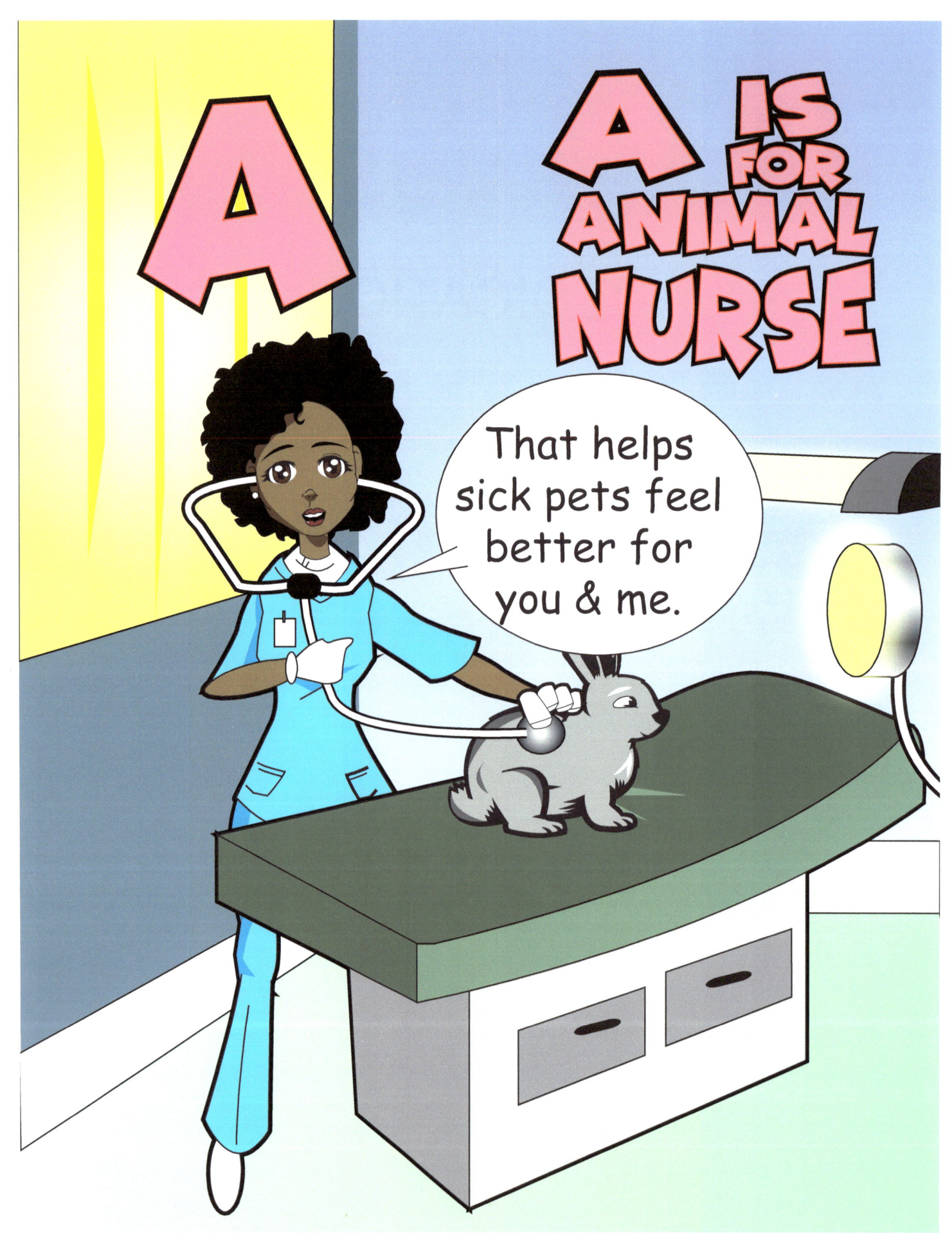

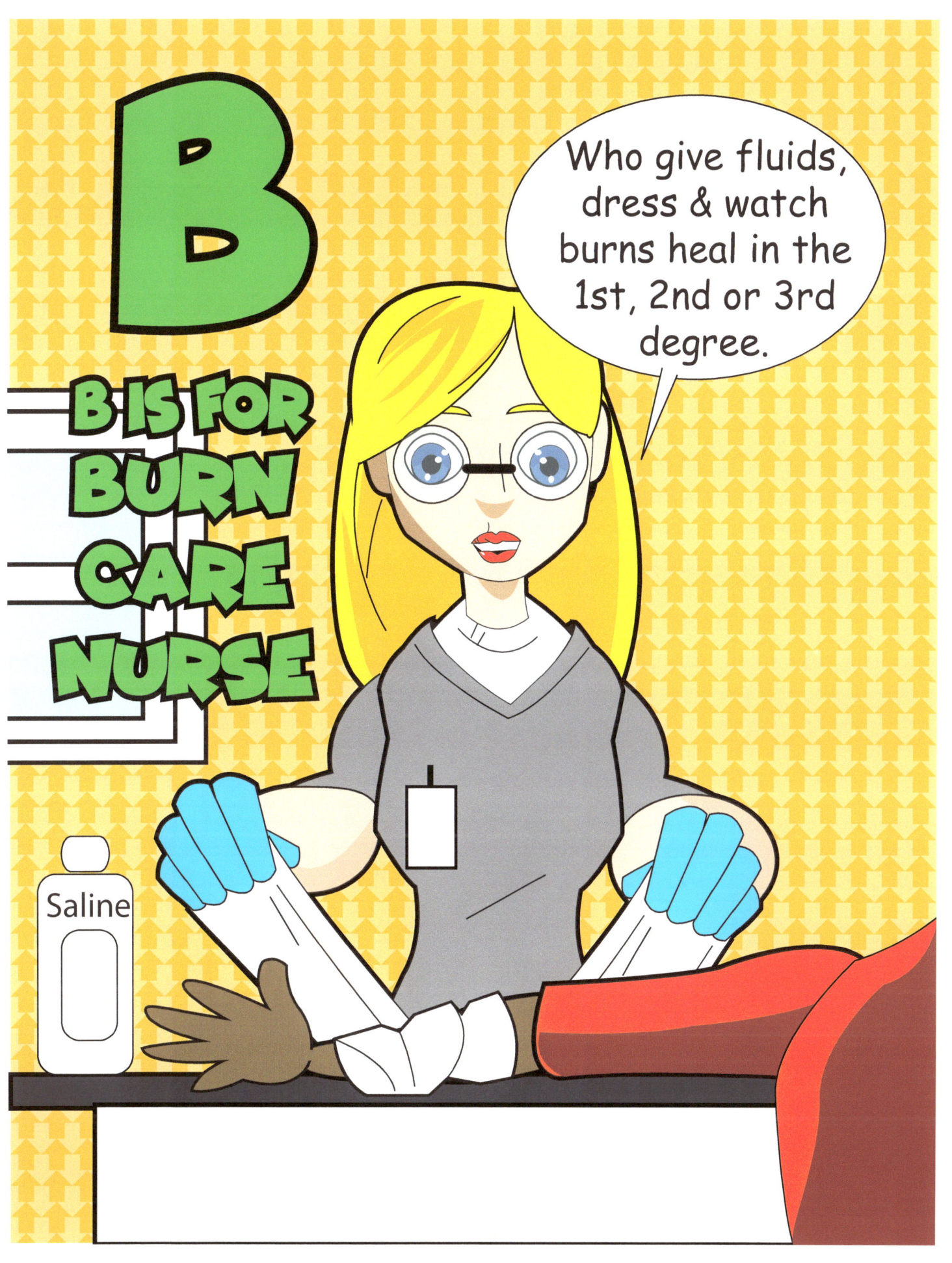

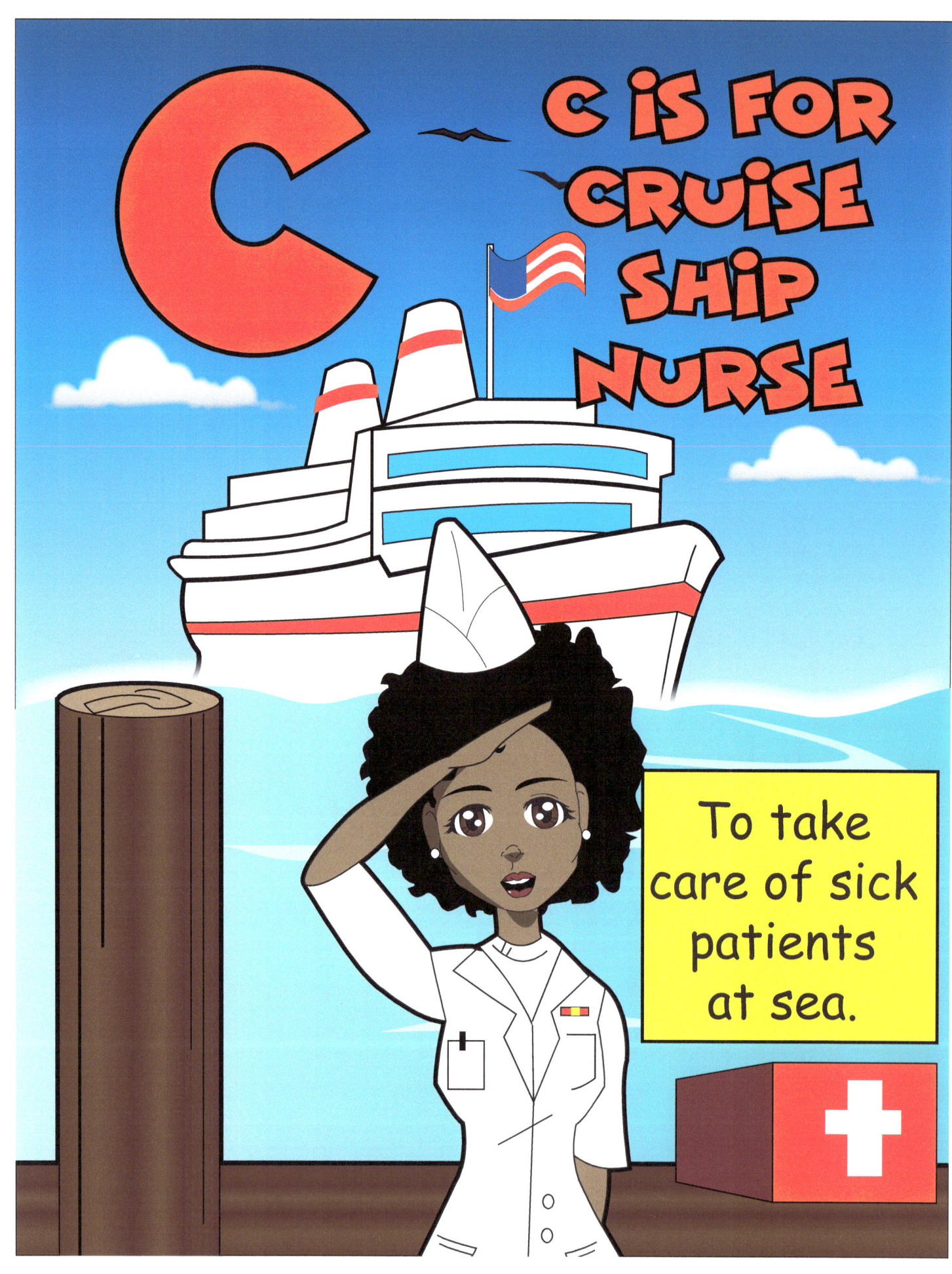

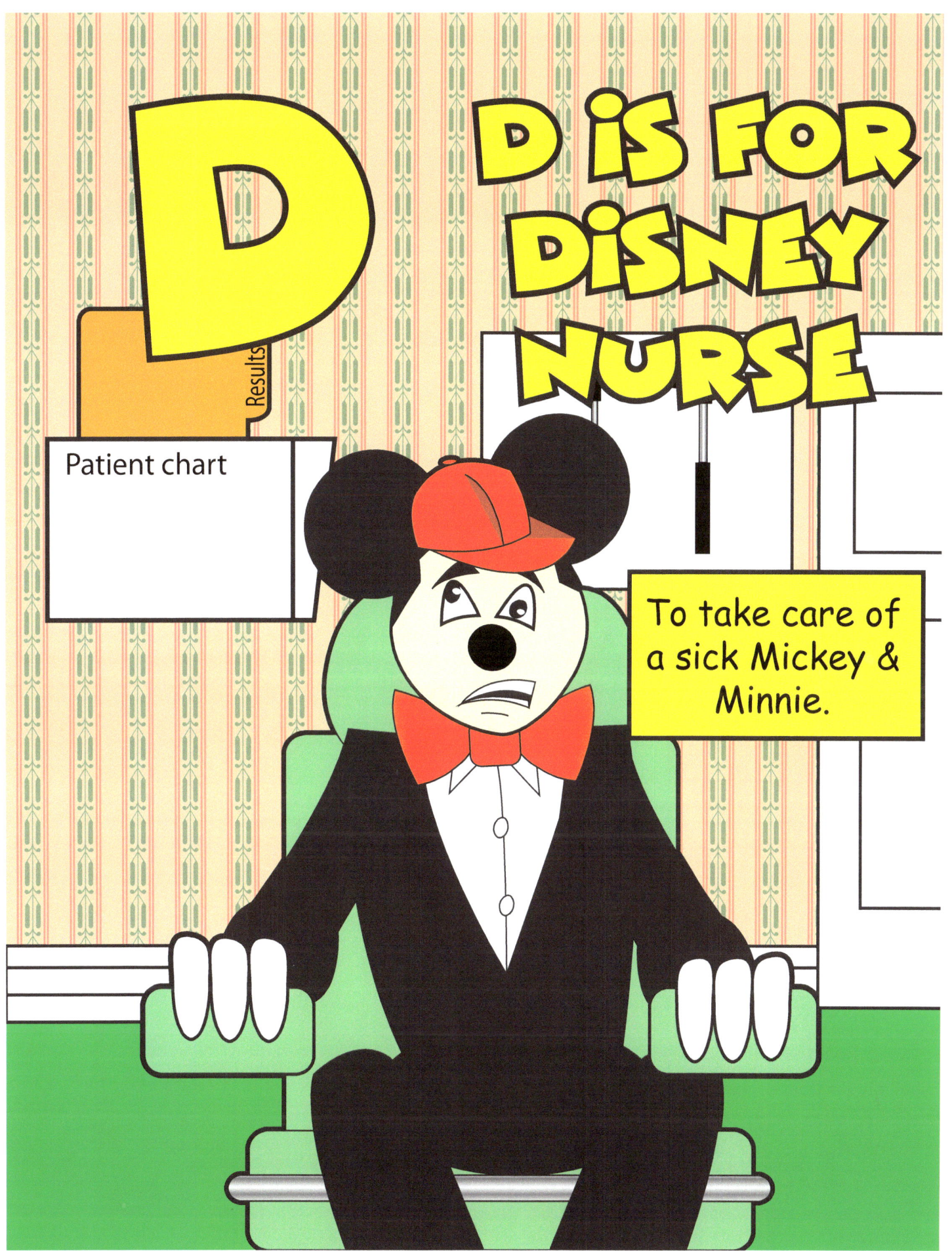

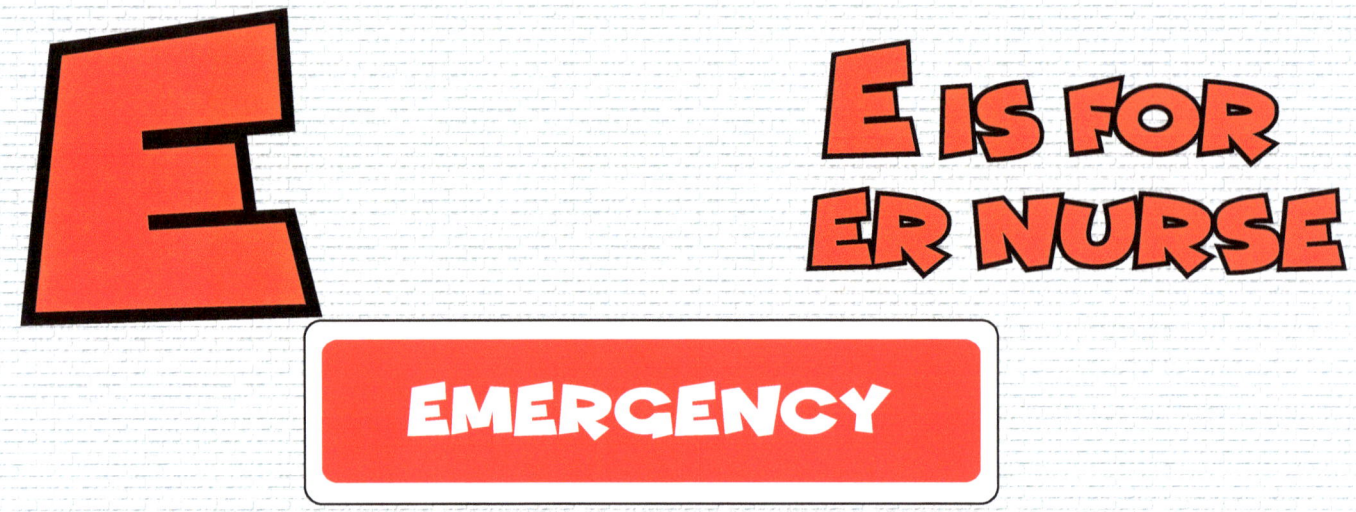

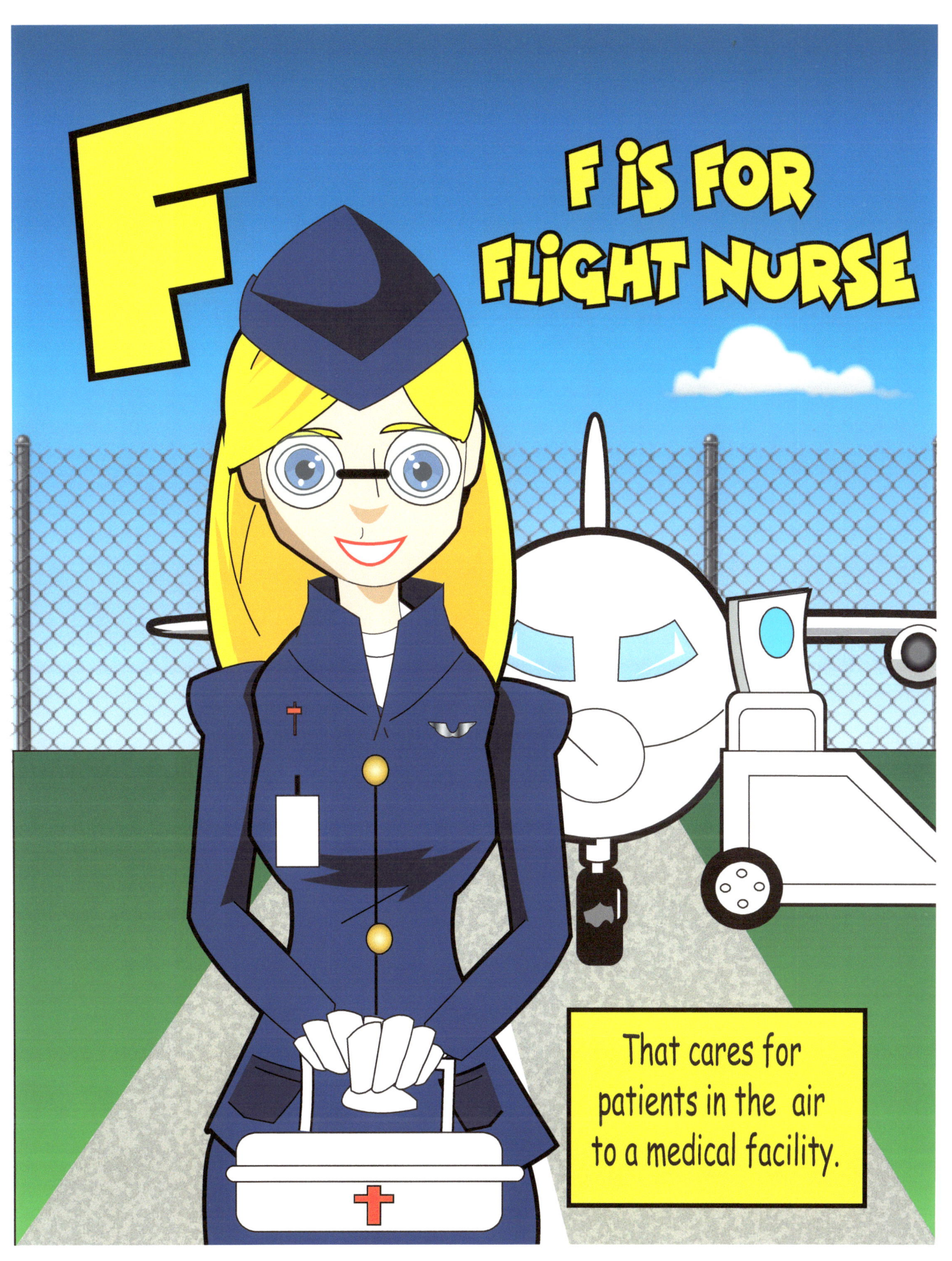

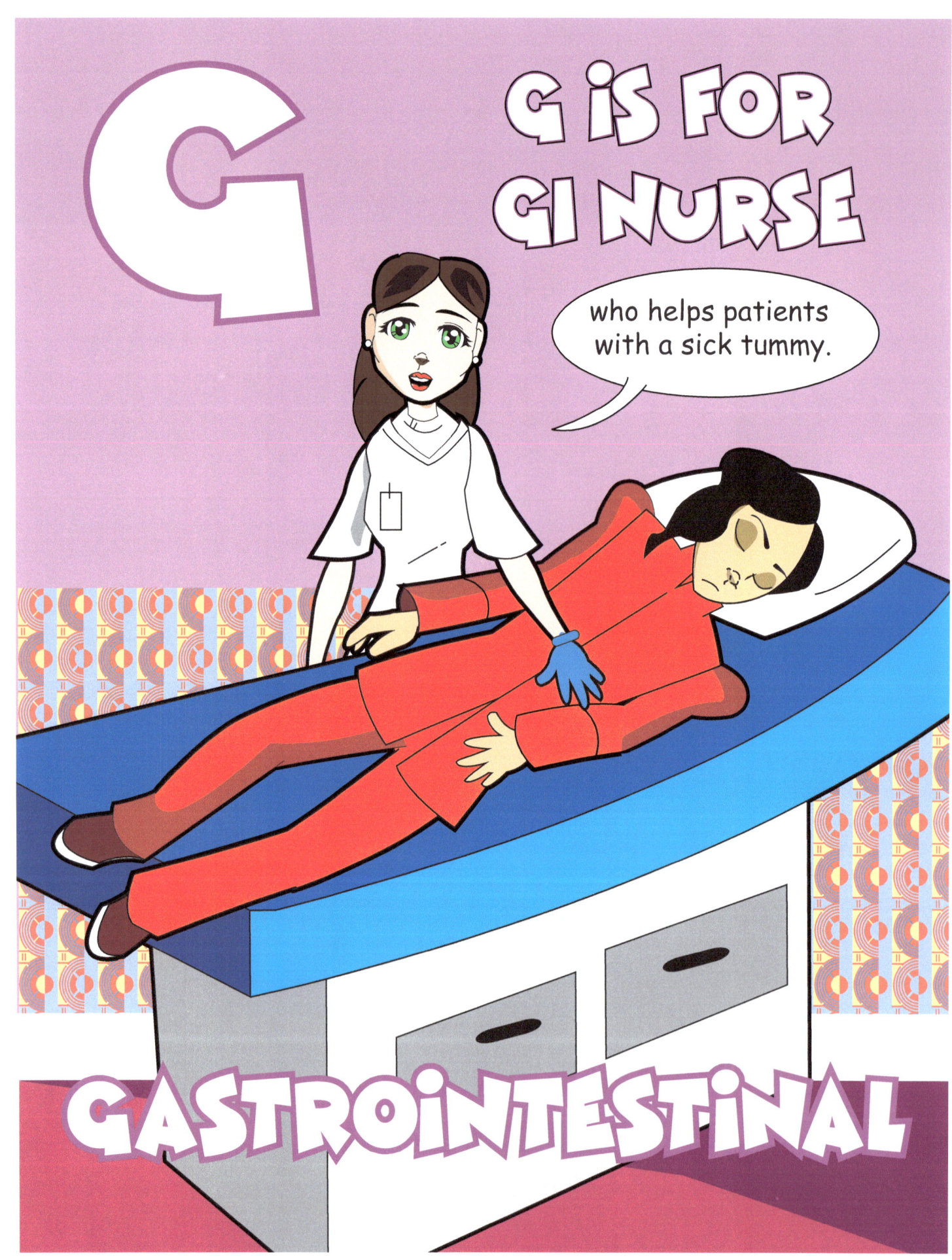

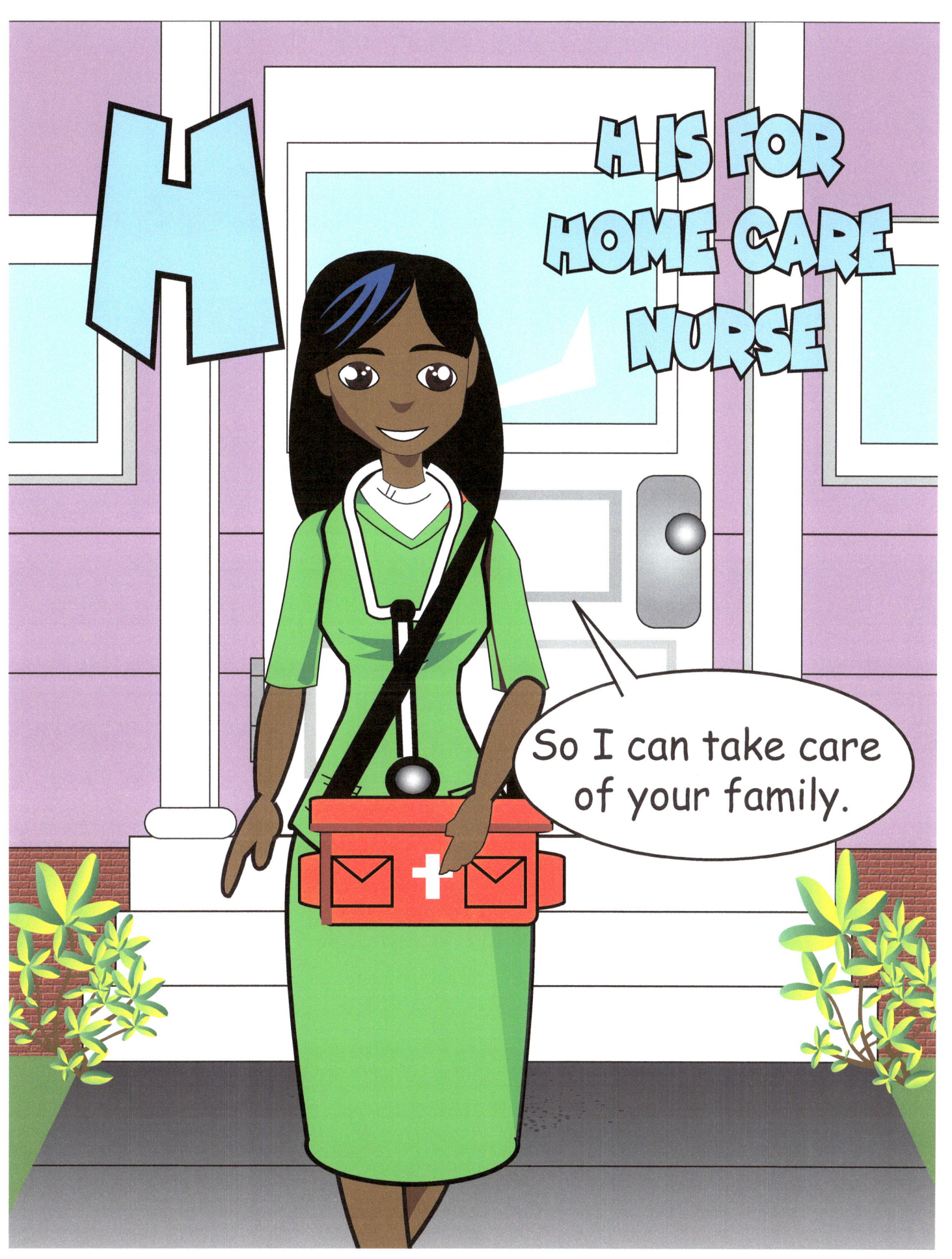

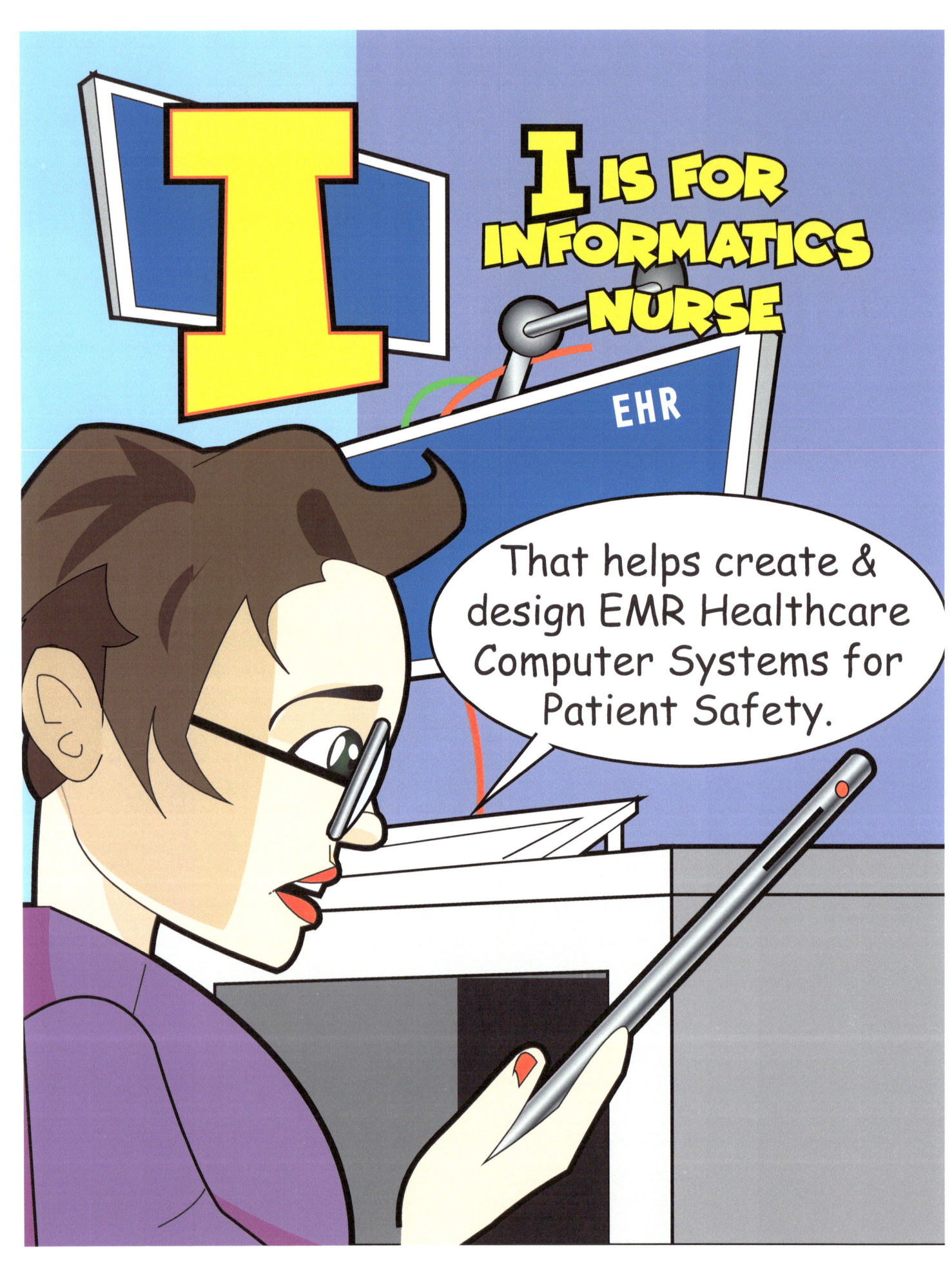

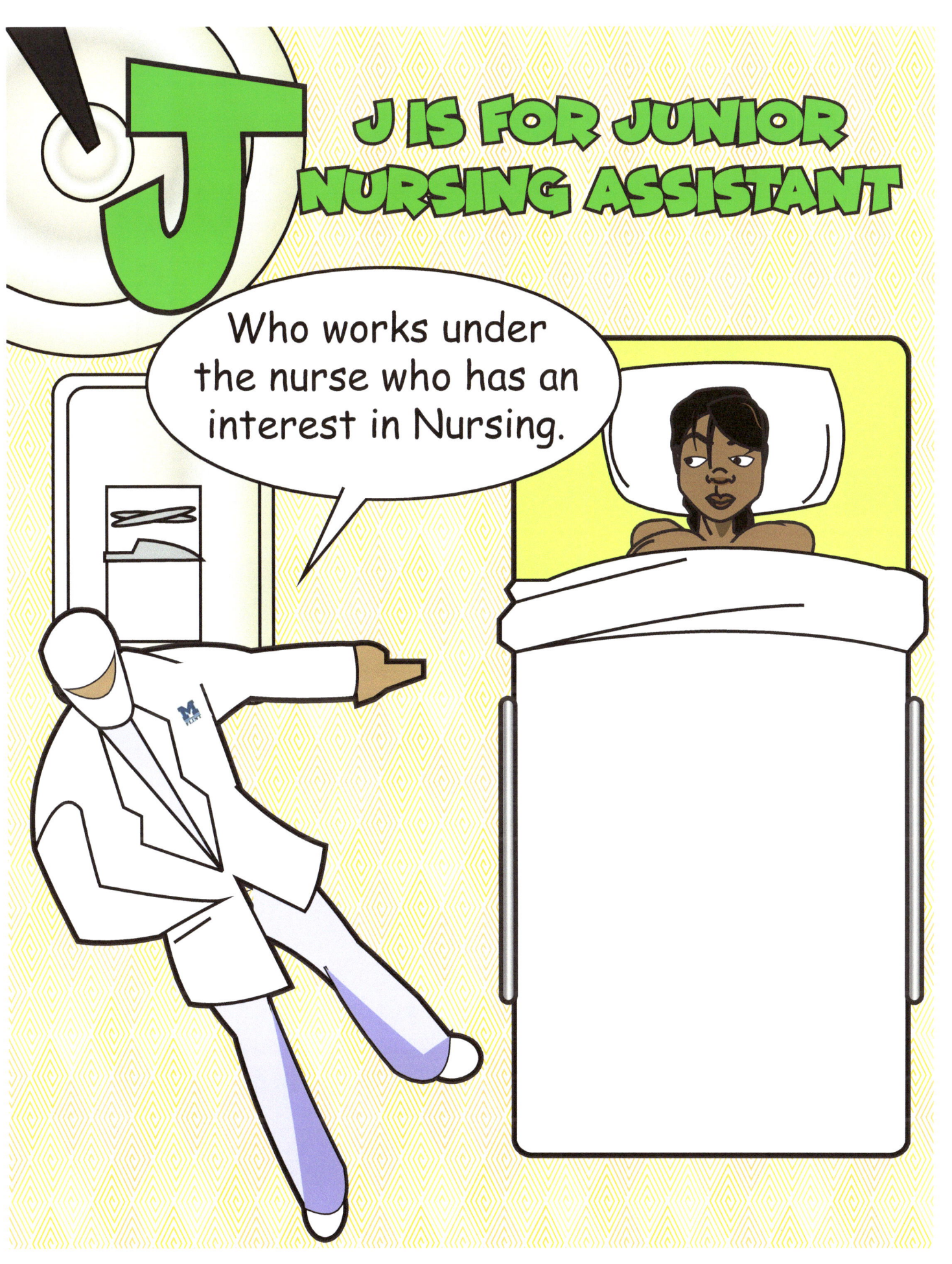

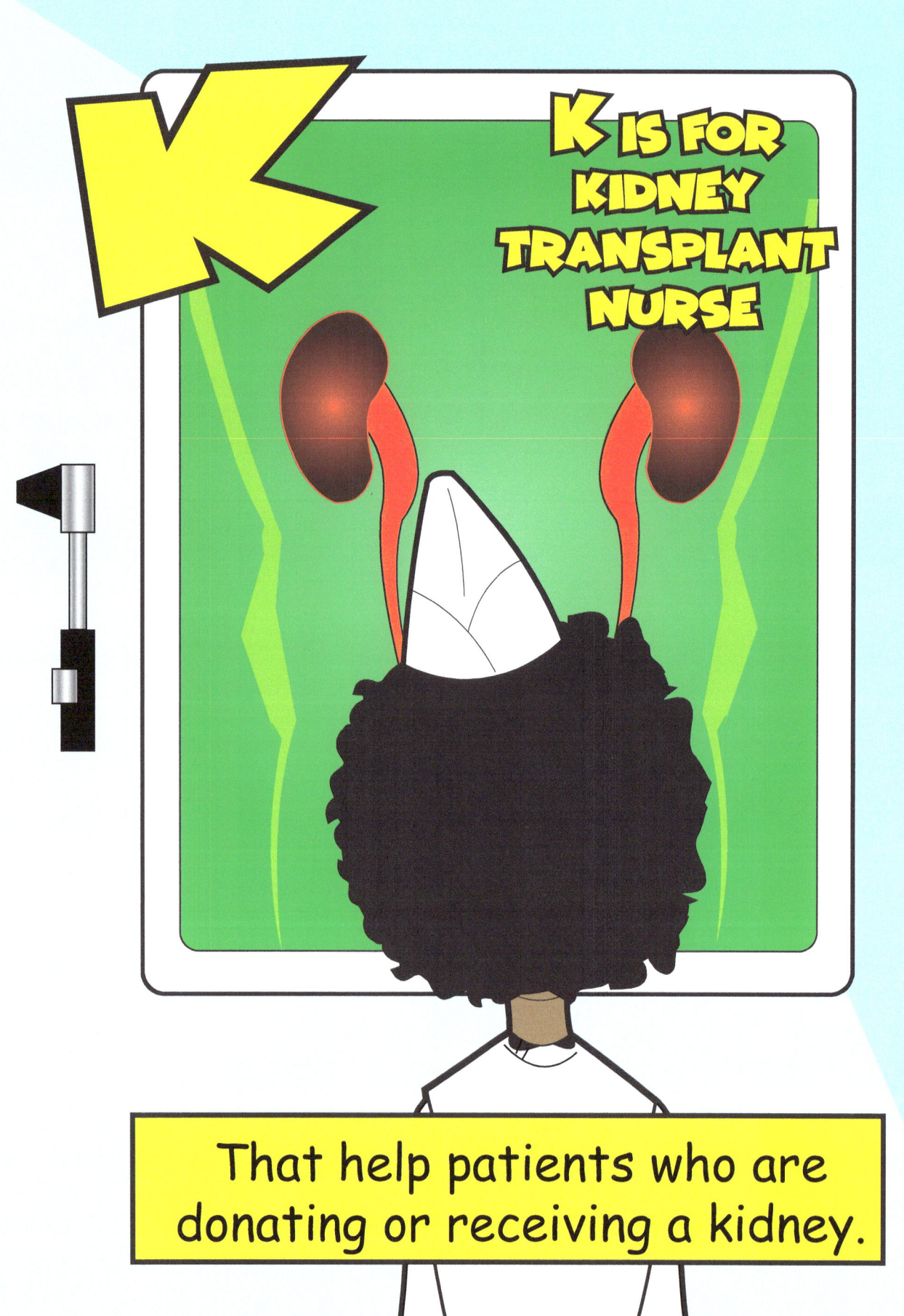

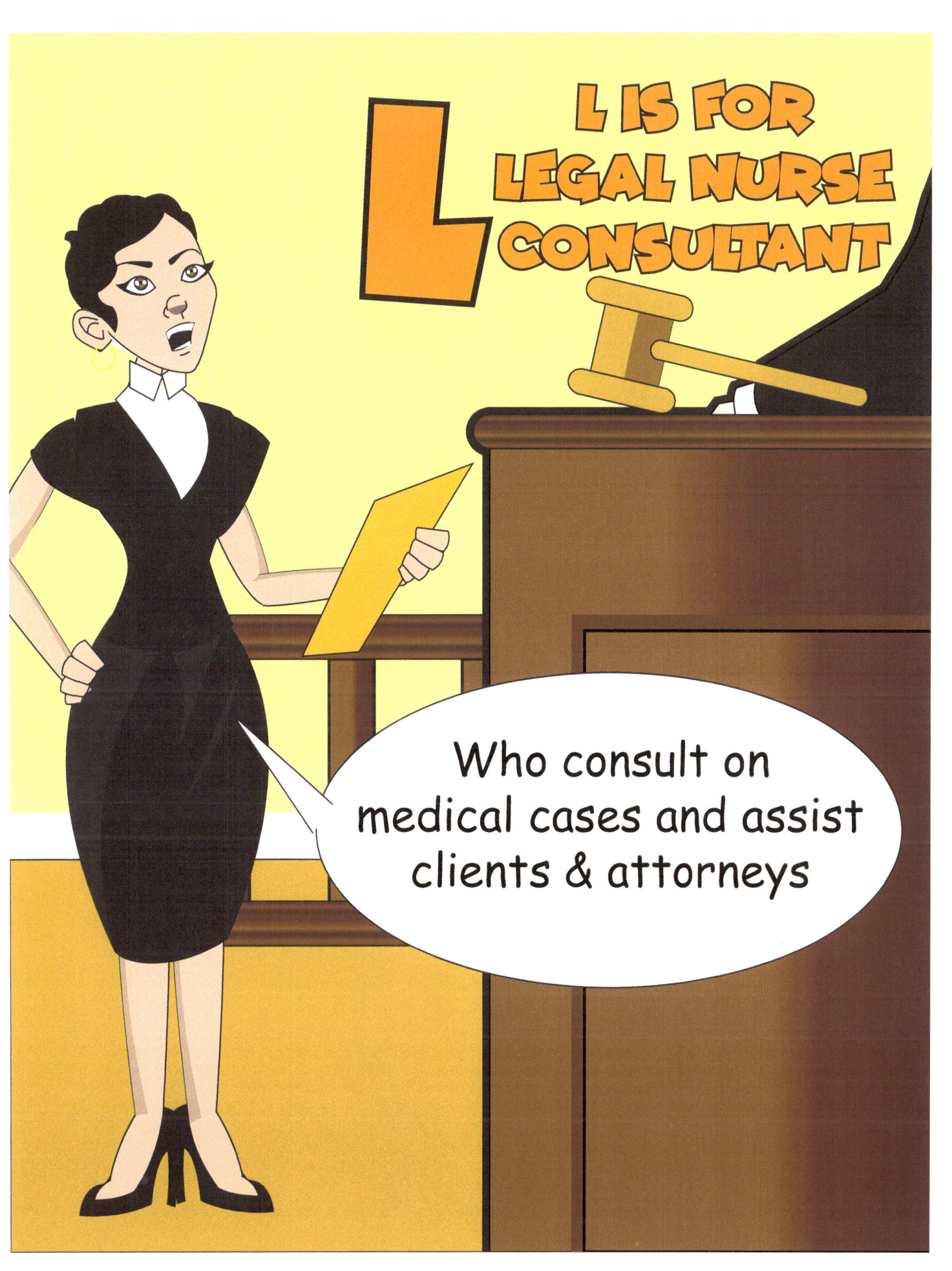

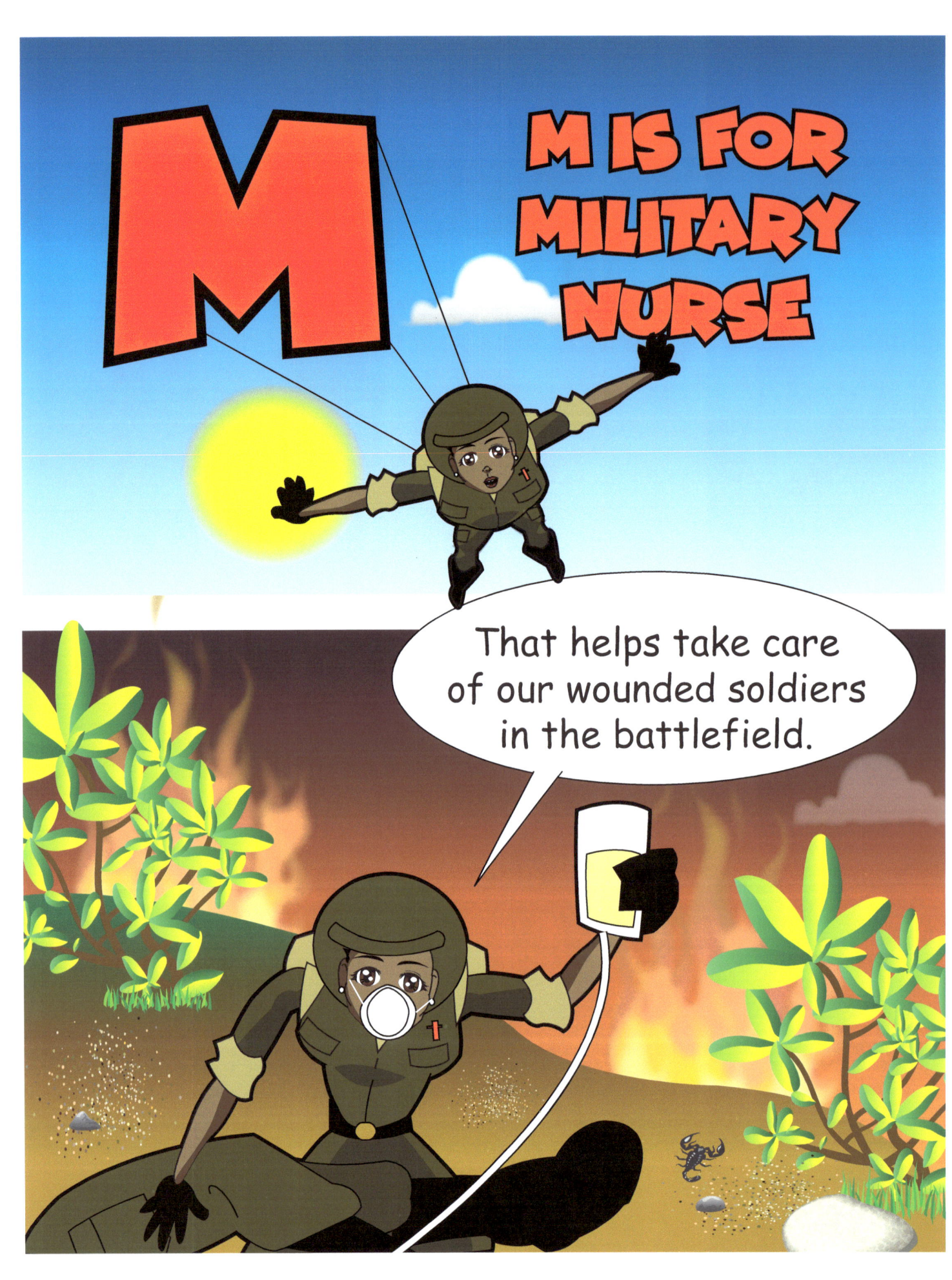

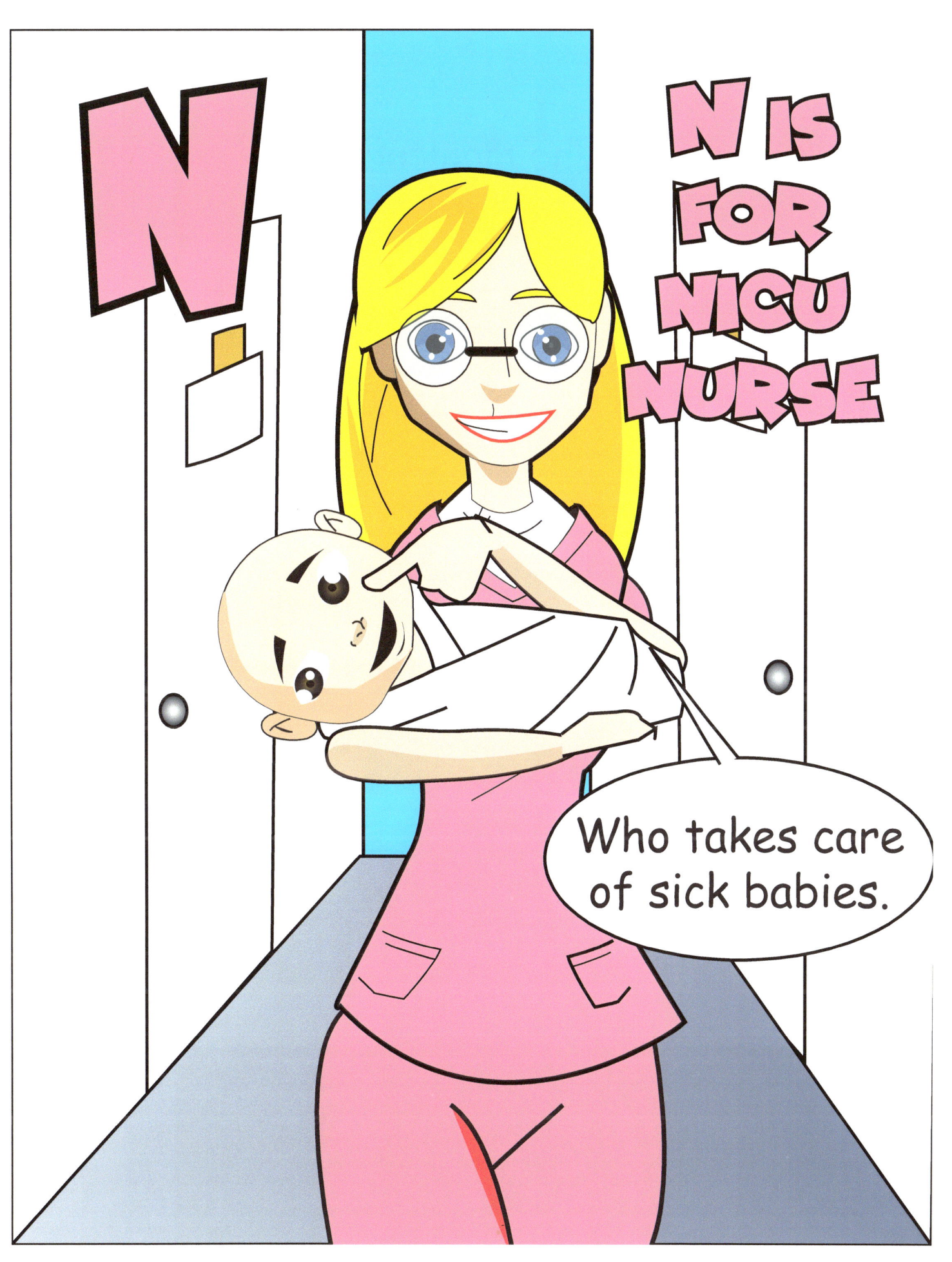

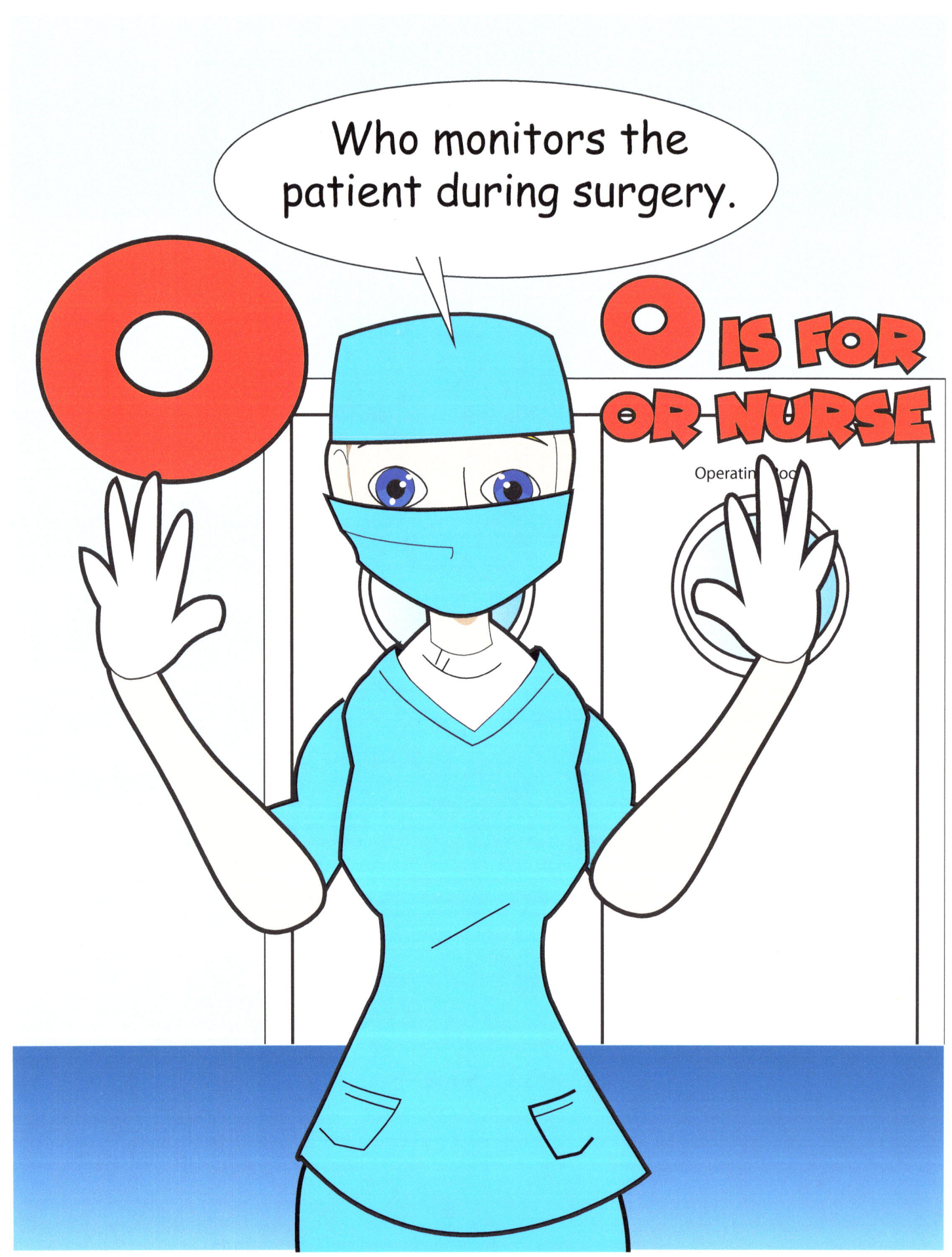

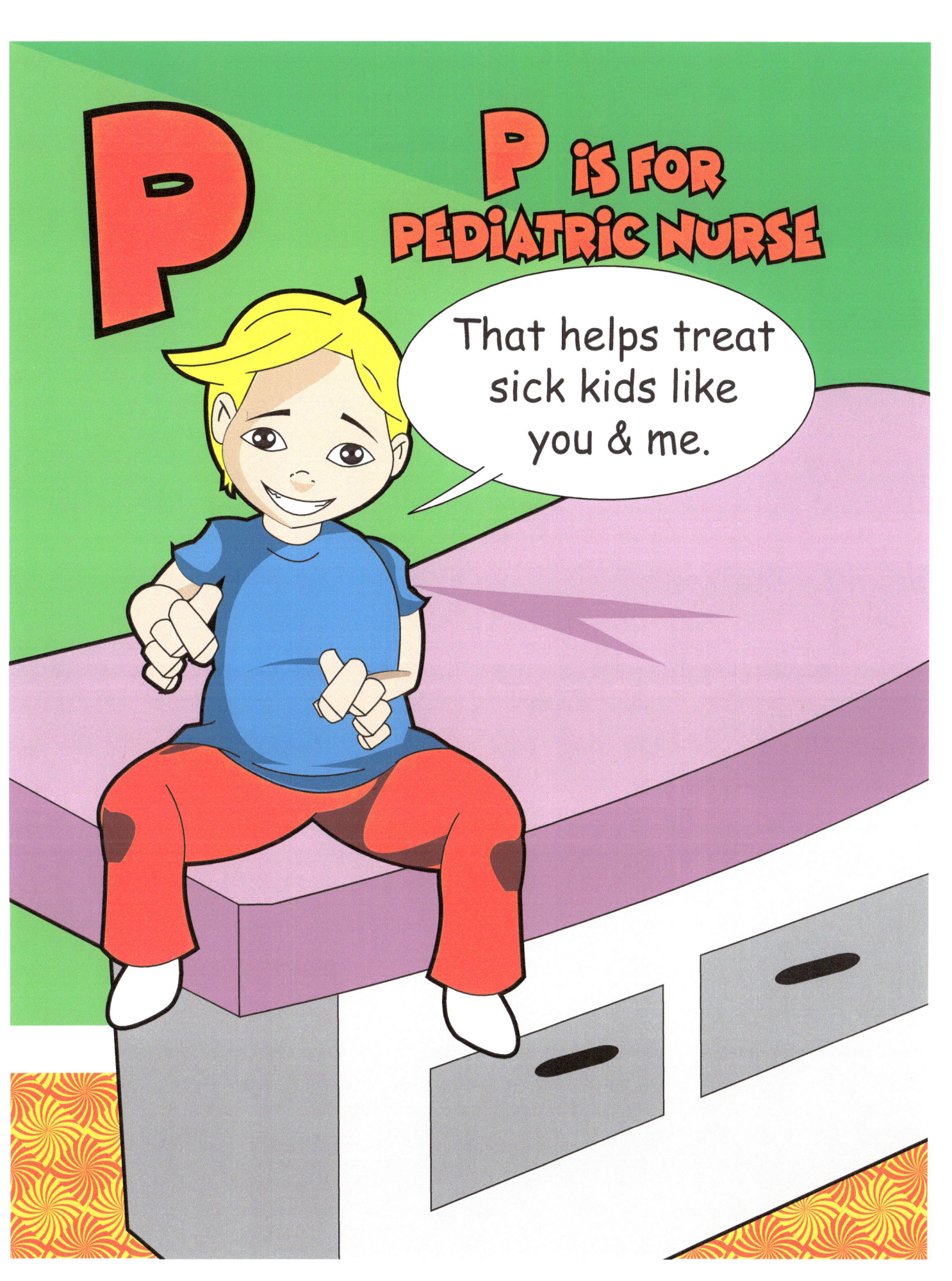

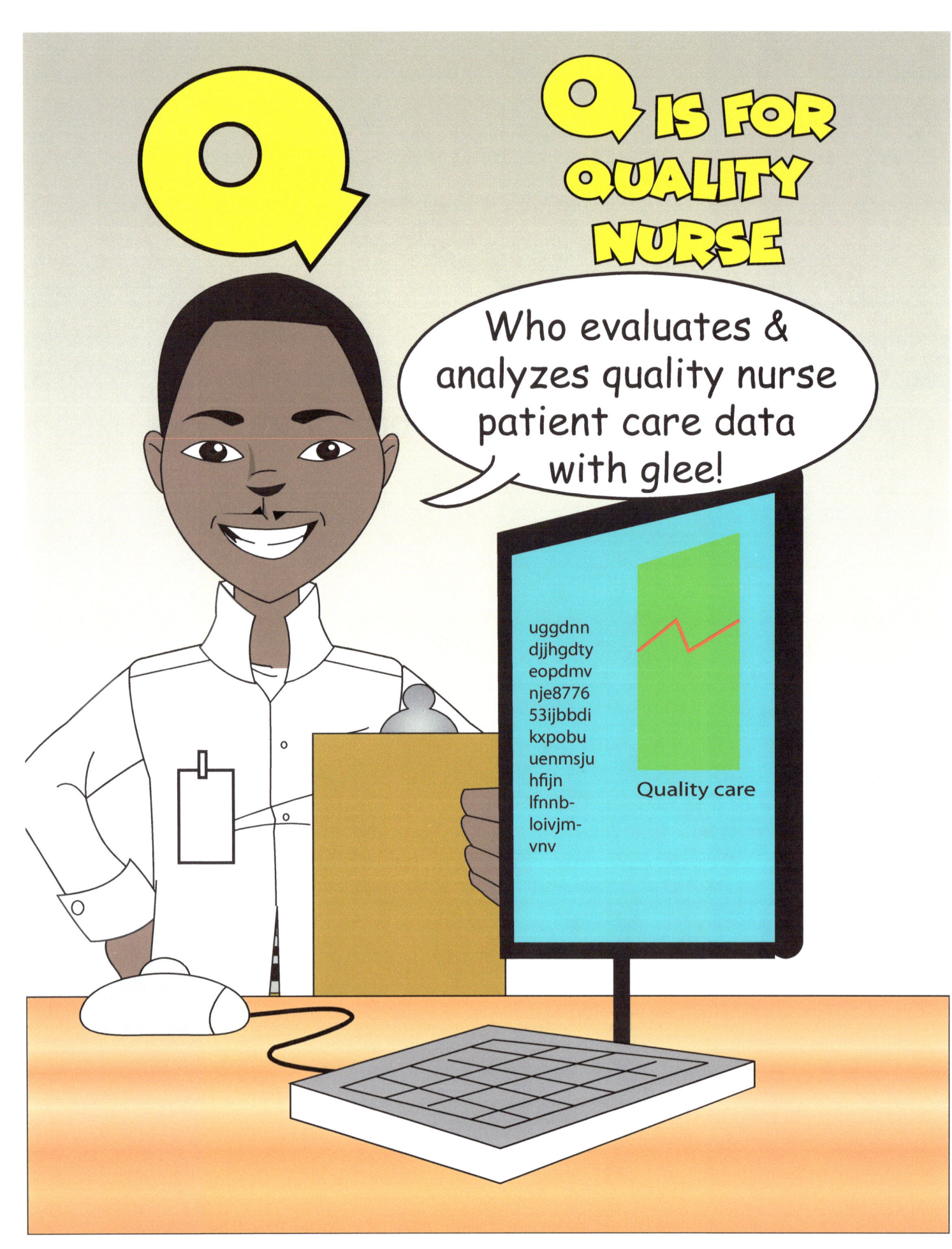

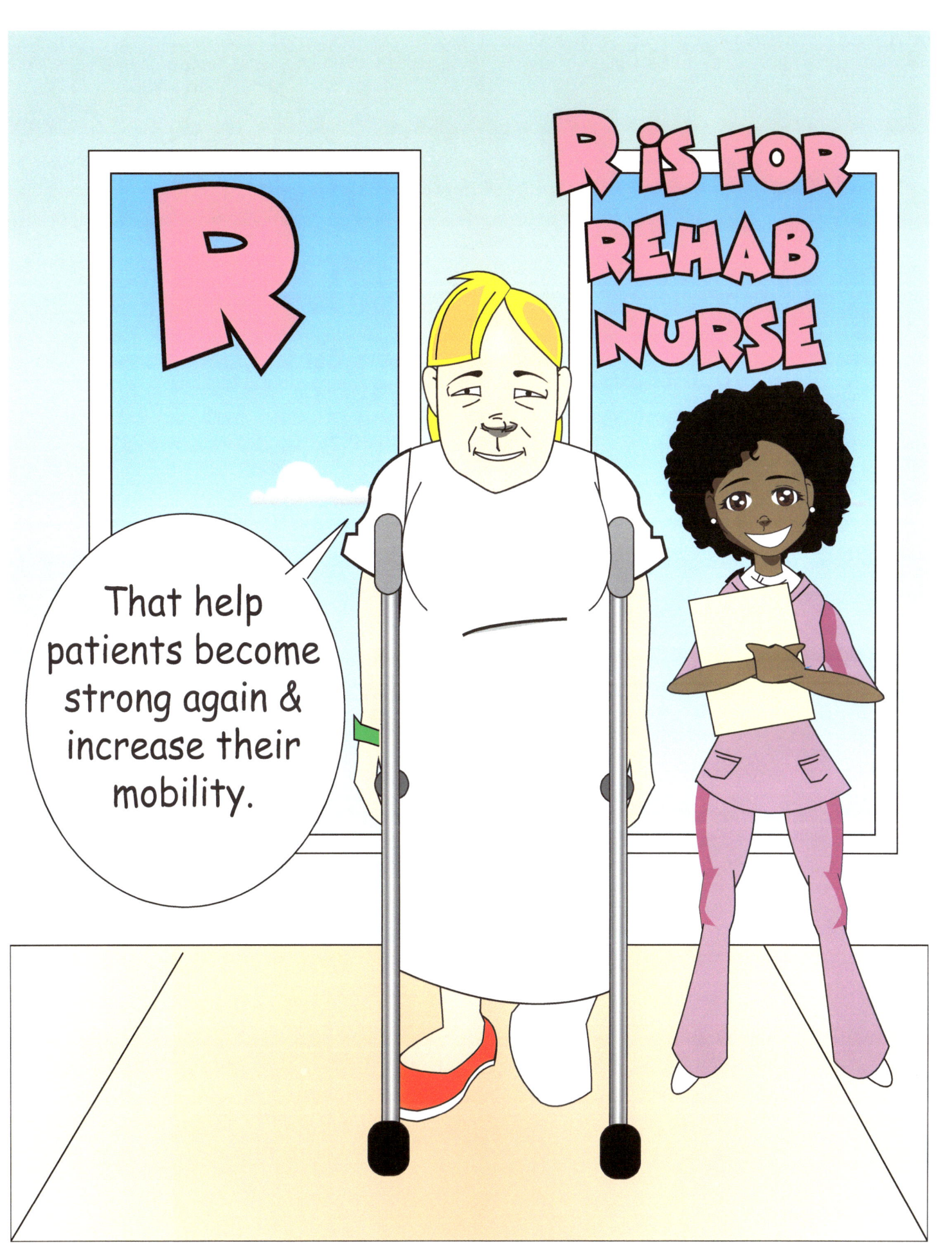

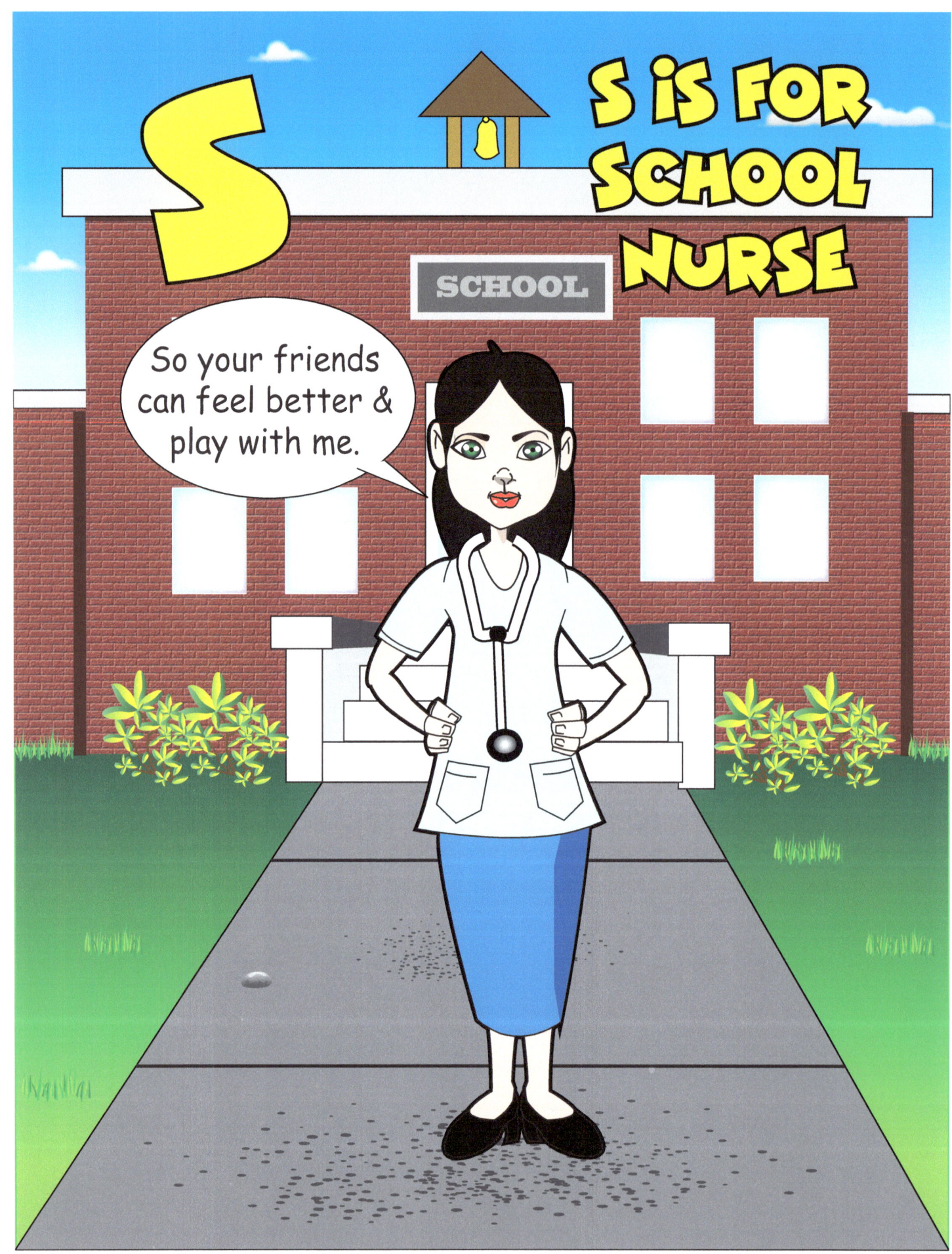

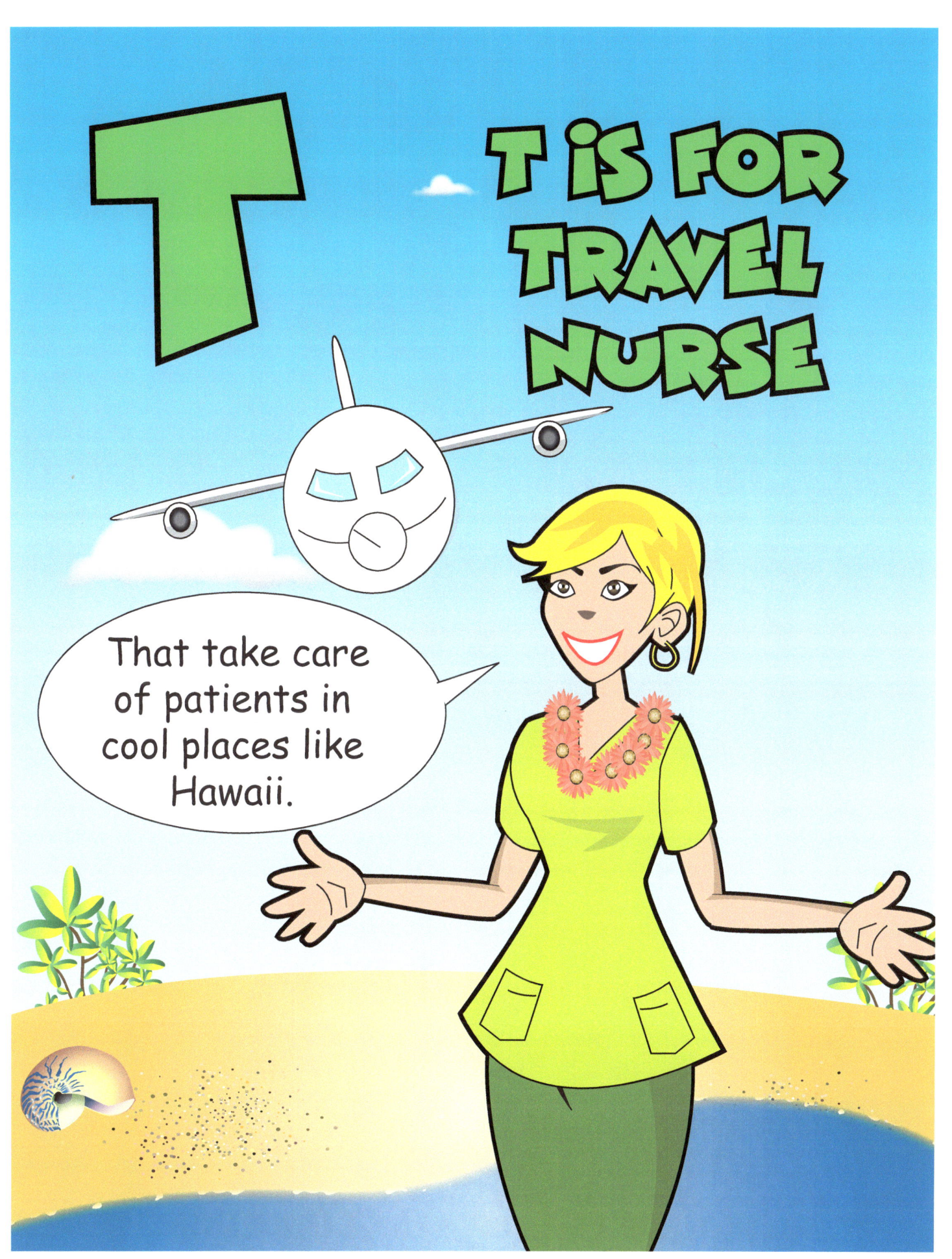

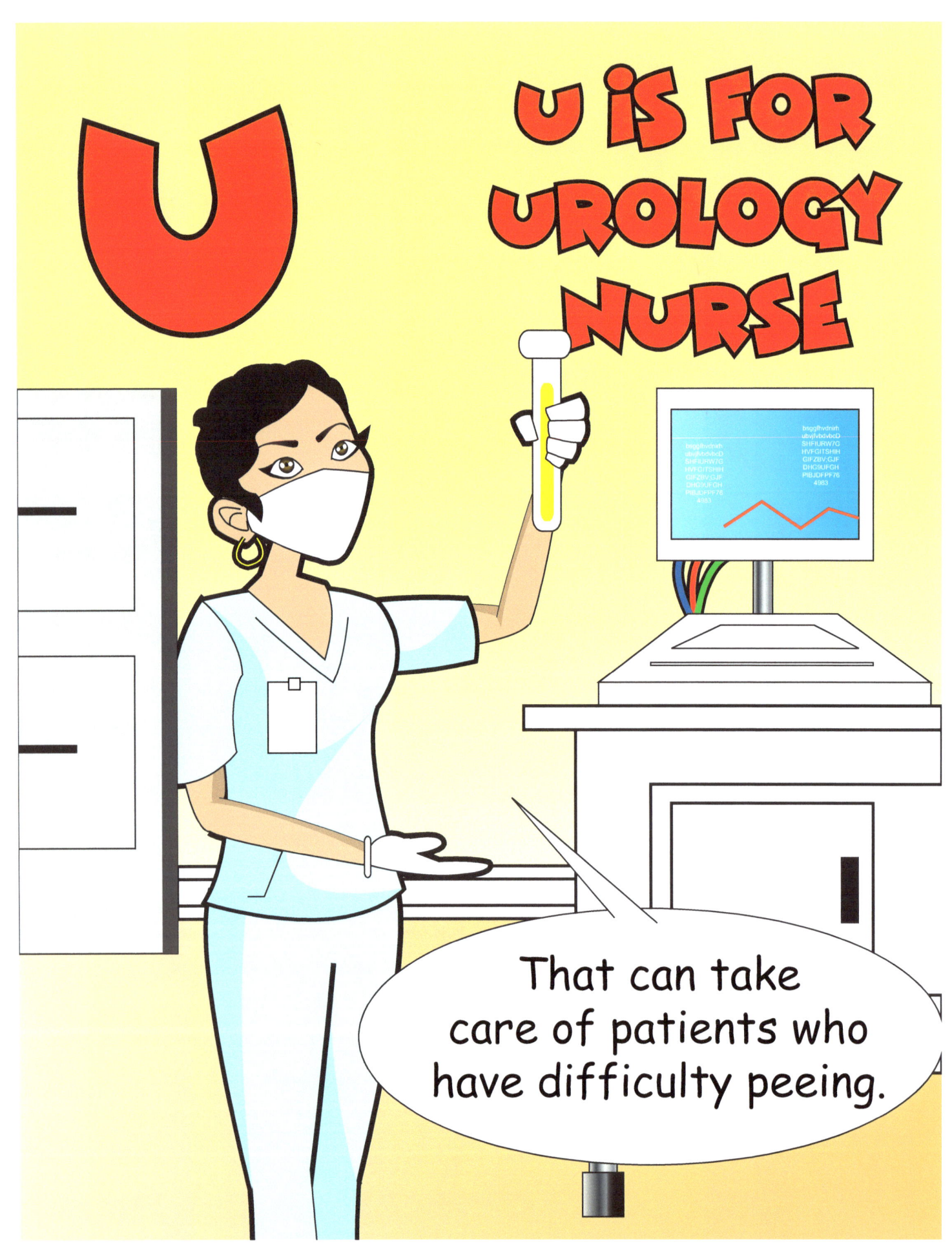

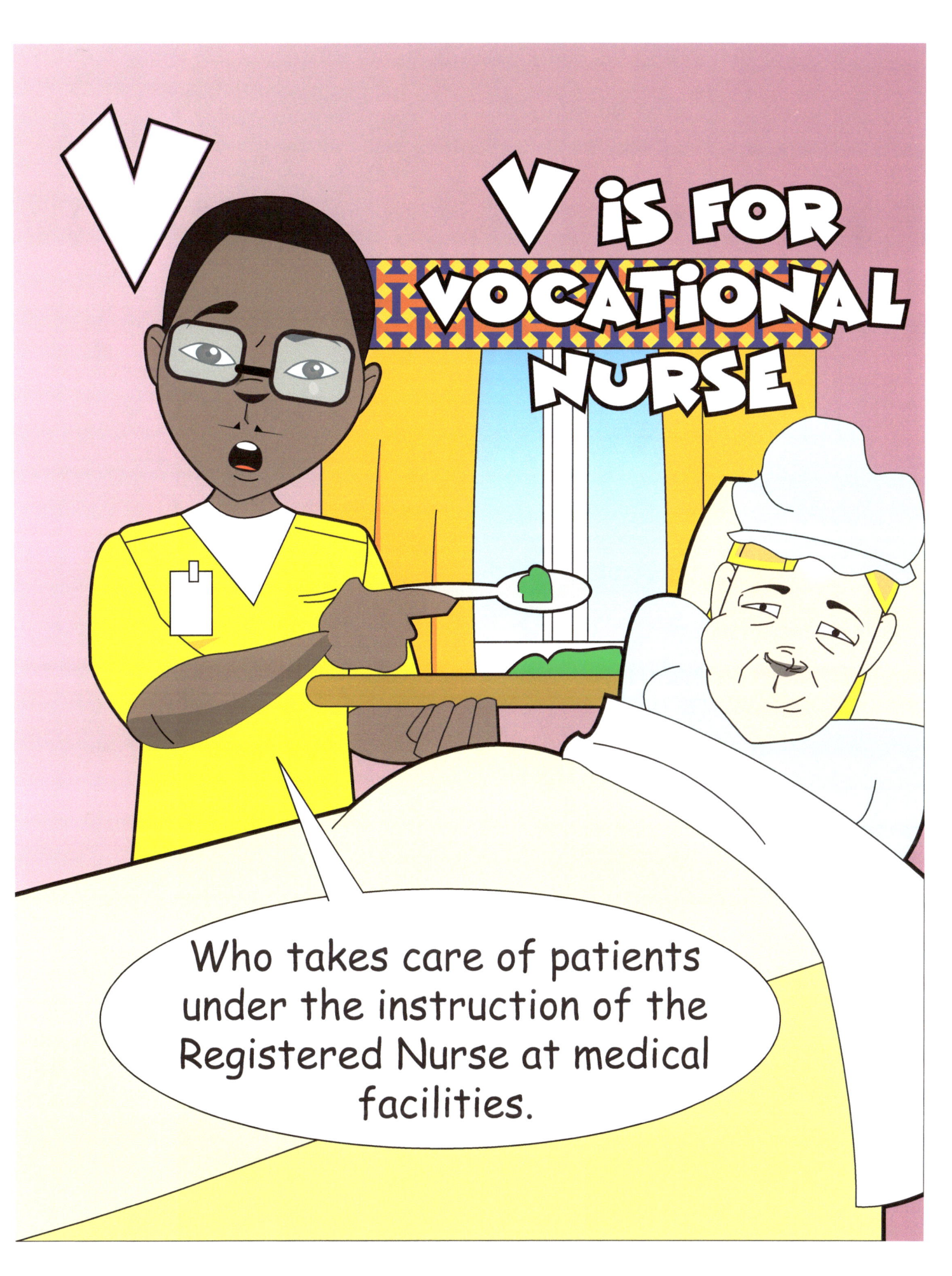

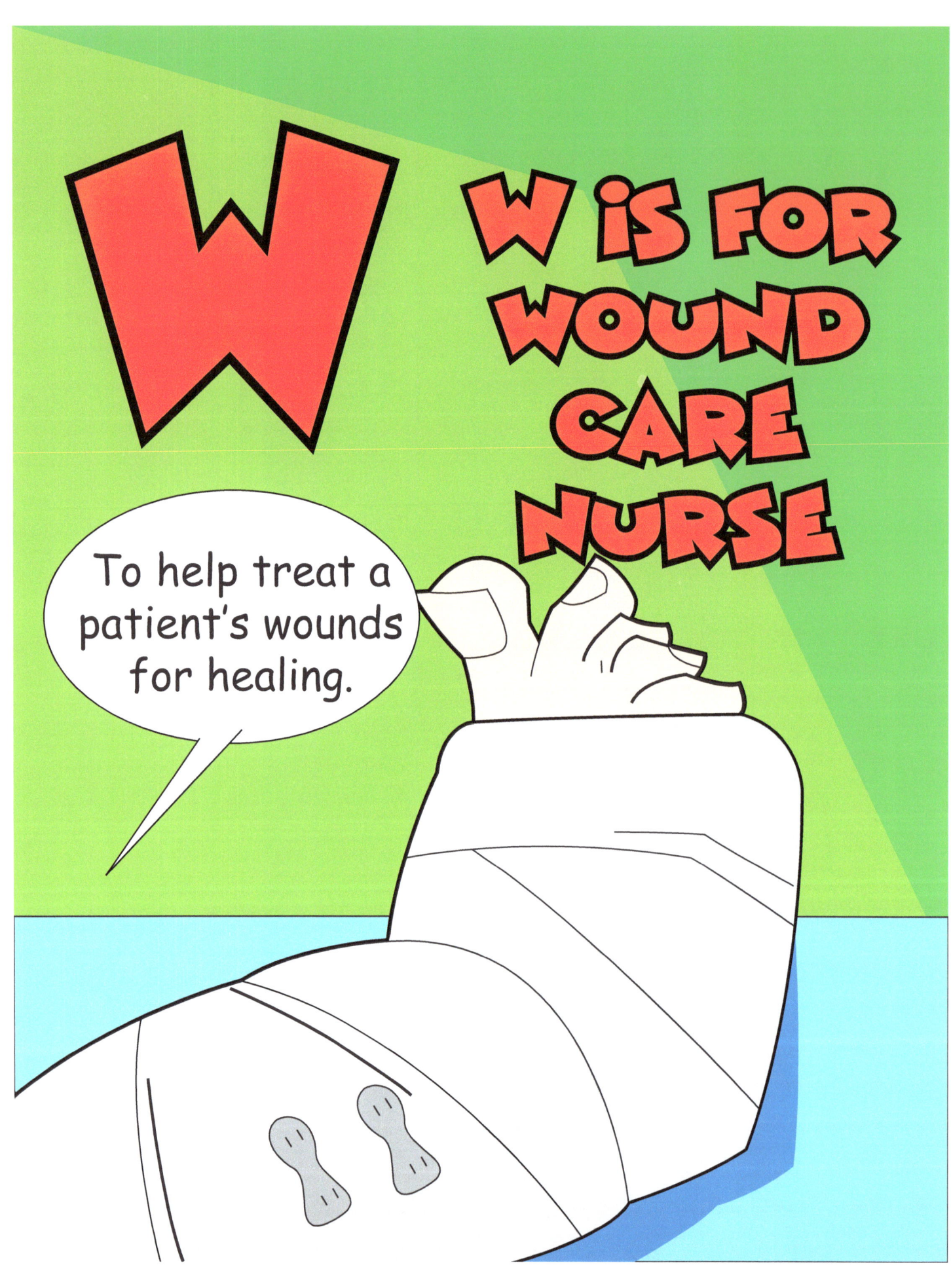

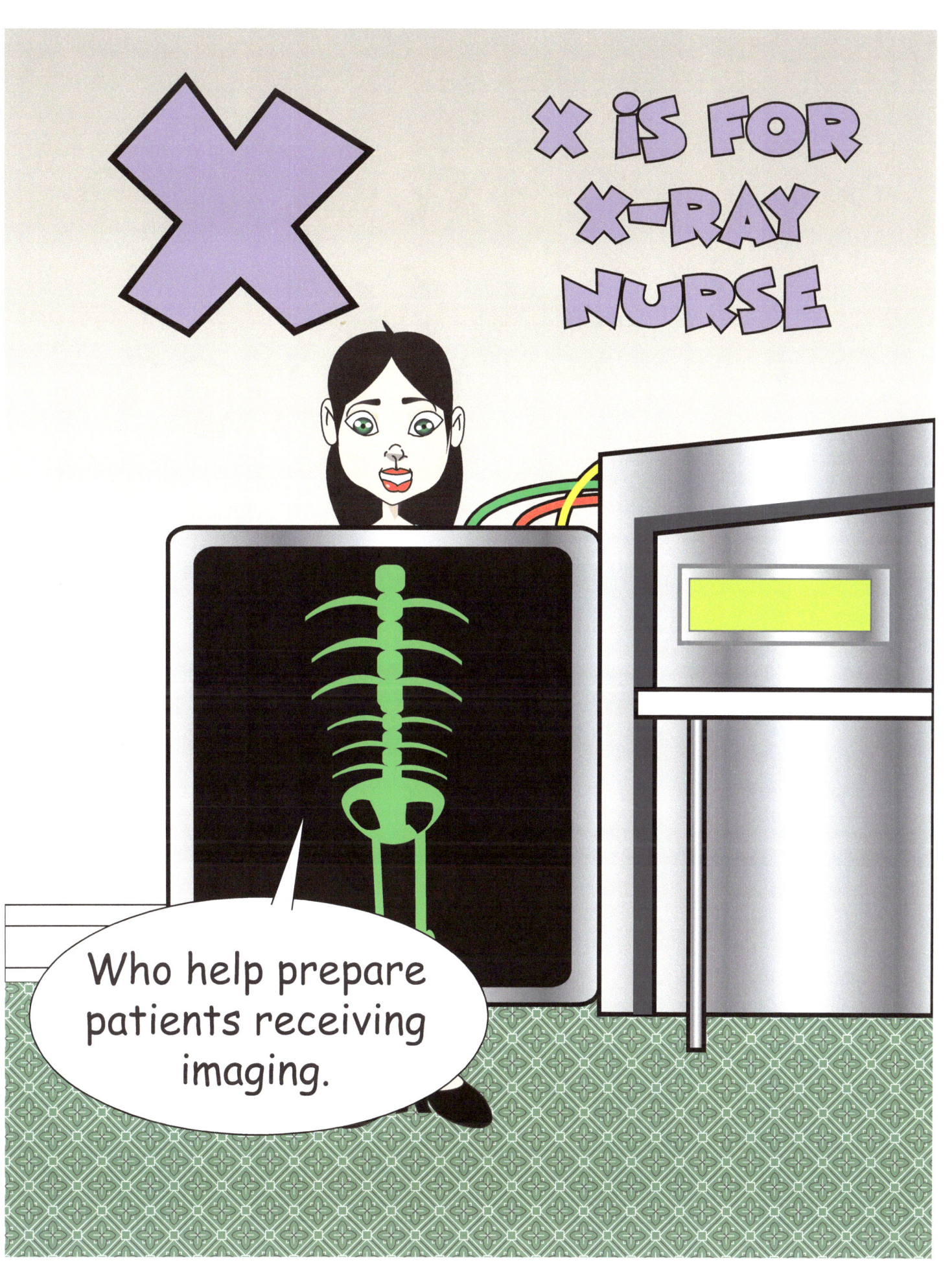

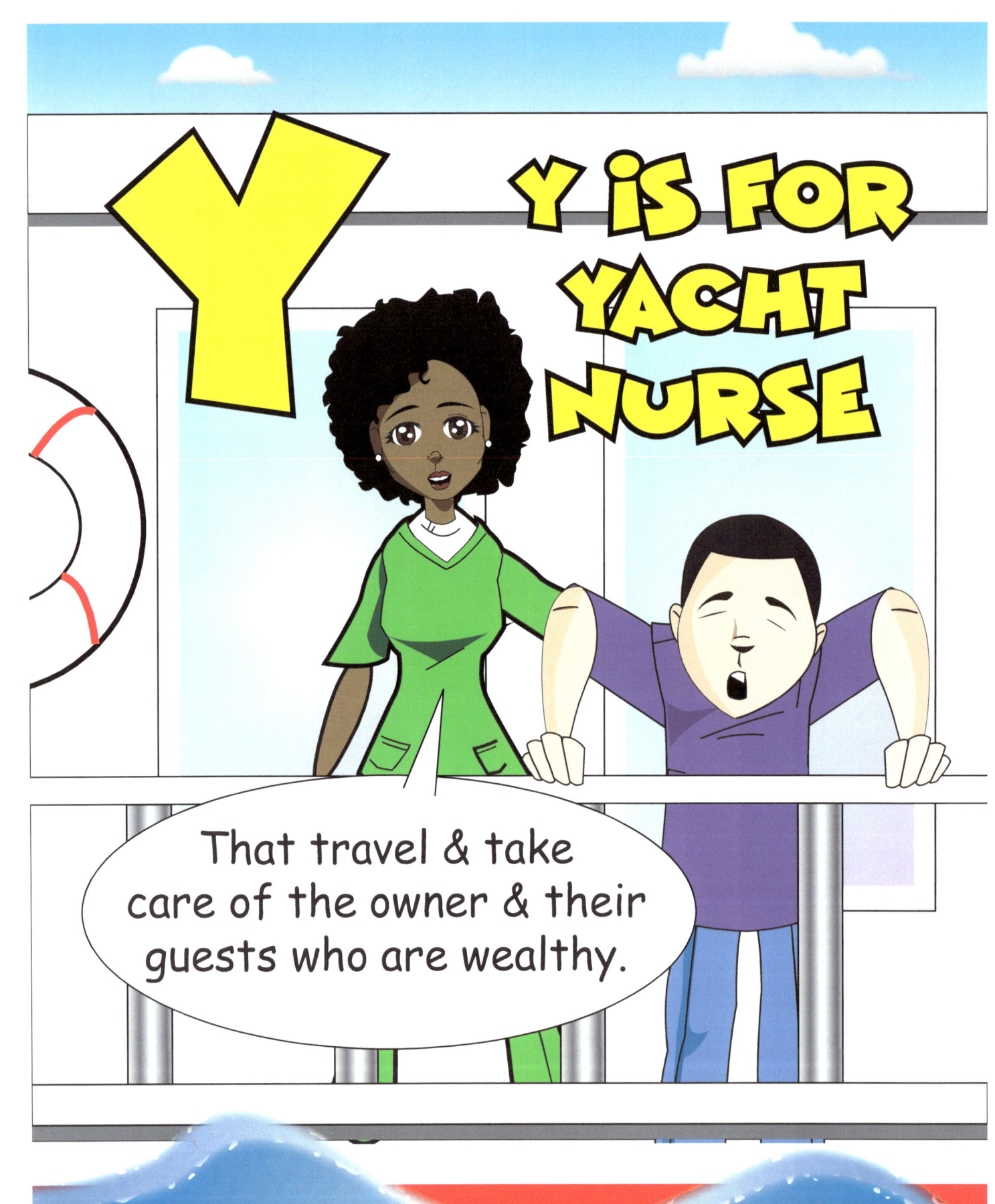

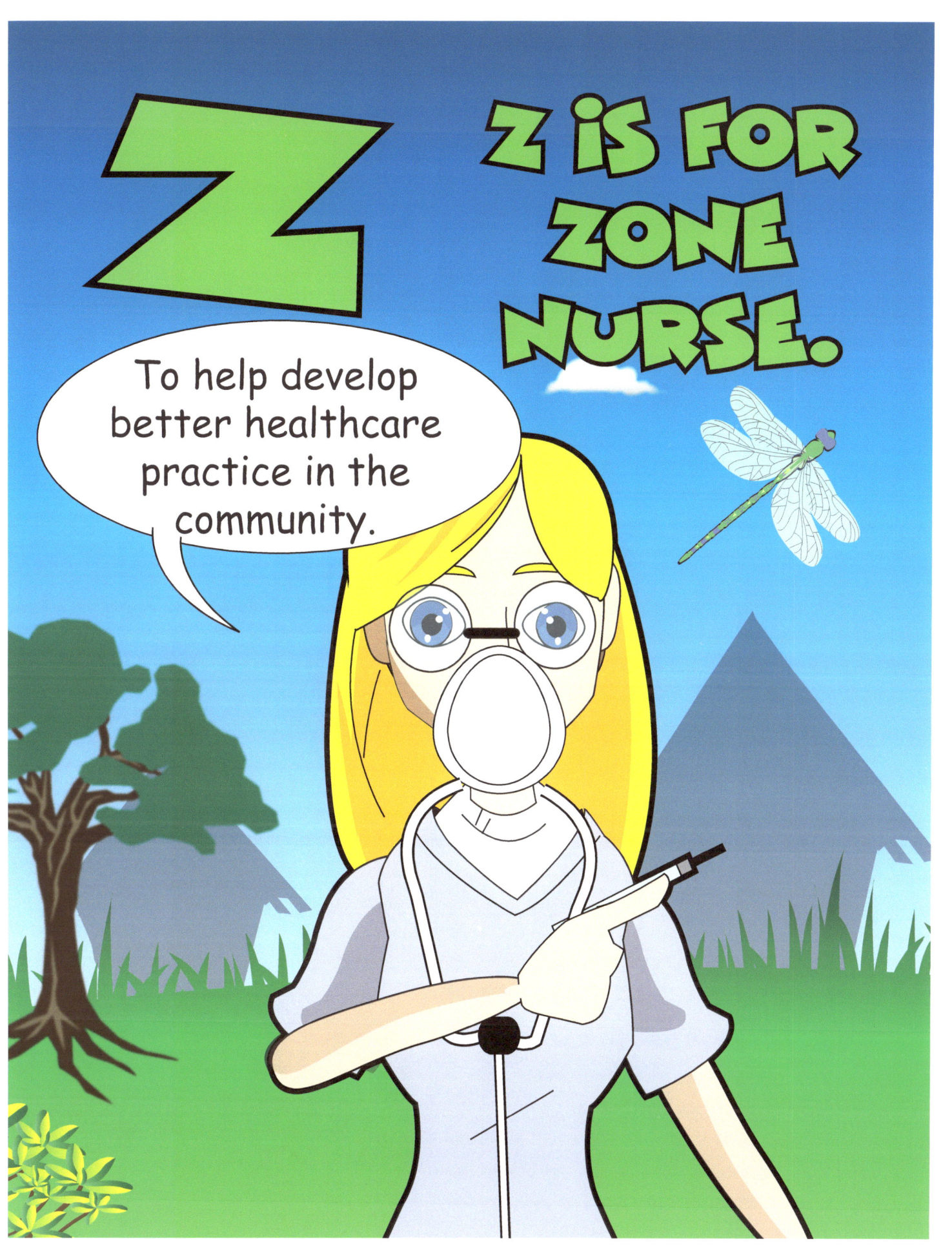

www.ingramcontent.com/pod-product-compliance
Lightning Source LLC
Chambersburg PA
CBHW040057250526
45473CB00043B/1814